108 Insights into

Tai Chi Chuan

D1374145

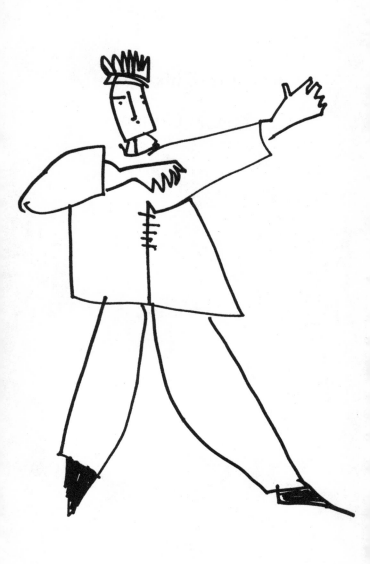

108 Insights into Tai Chi Chuan

A String of Pearls

Michael Gilman

YMAA Publication Center
Wolfeboro, NH

Publisher's Cataloging-in-Publication

(Provided by Quality Books, Inc.)

Gilman, Michael.
    108 insights into tai chi chuan : a string of pearls /
Michael Gilman. — 2nd ed.
    p. cm.
    ISBN: 1-886969-58-2

    1. T'ai chi chuan. 2. Meditation—Taoism. I. Title.
GV504.G55 1998   613.7'148
                                      QBI97-41604

YMAA Publication Center
Main Office:
    PO Box 480
    Wolfeboro, New Hampshire, 03894
    1-800-669-8892 • www.ymaa.com • info@ymaa.com

20200217

Printed in USA.

Dedicated to Dana Michelsen, without her loving support and encouragement this would not have been possible.

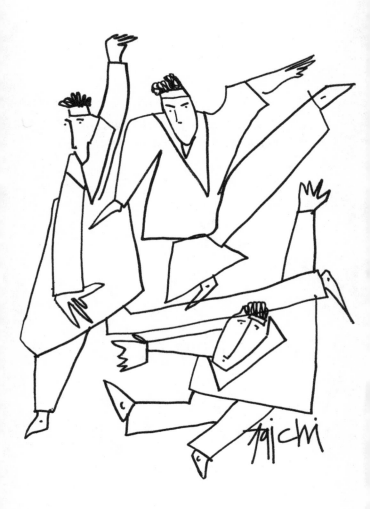

Introduction

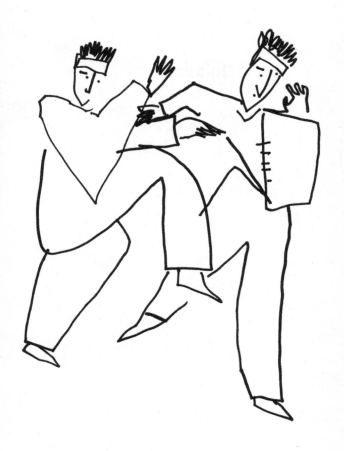

Tai Chi Chuan has been compared to a string of pearls. A pearl is formed by an oyster out of a need to deal with an irritating object. For humans, this irritation can have a physical, mental or spiritual basis, maybe all three. Tai Chi evolved, like a pearl, to deal with these irritations. A grain of sand is surrounded in defense by the oyster to form a smooth pearl. A threat or need to our individual self is made into a movement of such beauty by the Tai Chi principles that almost everybody feels a deep sense of awe. These separate moments are strung together to make Tai Chi Chuan, as practiced by most people today. In traditional Yang Style Tai Chi, according to customary counting, there are 108 movements, so I have decided to use 108 as my String of Pearls.

I have practiced Tai Chi Chuan since 1968, and have been teaching since 1973. I have studied with many teachers and read most of the books that have been written about Tai Chi. The wonderful thing about Tai

Chi is how universal a study it is. People from all over the world study and practice, and we could all be in the same place practicing and that would be our common bond. No words have to be exchanged, as Tai Chi is a physical art, a martial art, and a meditative moving art. There are no words that can possibly describe the actual movements, only hints to help you to get mind and body moving together.

There are quite a few books out, in fact most, that attempt to teach the Tai Chi movements. Could you read a book to learn to walk if you had never seen walking? Or dance, swim, or ride a bike? As far as I know, it has never been done. Once you know how to walk, dance, swim, or ride, a book can be helpful to explain how others go about the same activities, what they think about when engaging in that move. To be in the presence of one who is truly accomplished in any activity is a rare event, not available to most of us. So books are helpful. They allow one person to talk to many and share what they think, feel and experience. It is not the same as being able to do Tai Chi with a master, yet it is an aid.

What I've tried to do in this little book is share with the reader some of my ideas and experiences that have evolved out of almost 30 years of consistent Tai Chi study and practice. I cannot say all these ideas are originate with me. I don't know where they come from. The Classic teachings of Tai Chi have been passed down for hundreds of years and, as each person digests the information, it gets passed to someone else in a slightly different way. In the United States, we understand images in a different way than the Chinese or Russians. I am a product of growing up in San Francisco during the 50's and 60's, and hopefully my words will be understandable to people with similar backgrounds. I want to pay special thanks and respects to the major influence in my Tai Chi career, and that is Master Choy Kam-Man. A quiet, gentle man who came to the U.S. from Canton, China, Master Choy helped me and innumerable others to begin to gain an understanding of Tai Chi. His whole life was devoted to teaching Tai Chi, and when unable to teach anymore because of illness, he let himself die in 1994. My last meeting with him was in 1993. I hadn't seen him for quite a few years. I had heard he wasn't well as he suffered from diabetes and was even on kidney dialysis. When I walked into his room, I was saddened to see him asleep in a chair, covered by a blanket. His hair was white, and his breathing shallow. He did not look well. His wife woke him up to announce my presence. It took him a while to gain enough energy to sit up, remove the blanket, get his glasses on, and bring me into focus.

Throughout all of this, many thoughts went through my head, the strongest being sadness. I realize that life comes and goes, yet we hate to let go of things that are important to us. My image of Master Choy was based on our interaction of years ago when he helped lift me onto my feet and head me on the road to health and happiness. I didn't know that our roles would be reversed, if only for a short time.

When he recognized me he started to perk up a bit. We chatted about why I was in San Francisco and things like that. When the subject got around to Tai Chi, his energy really started to move. He sat up straight and got excited as I told him about my classes and what I was working on at the time.

When the subject turned to Chi Kung, he got out of his chair and started to demonstrate what he was talking about. The transformation was complete. From hardly alive to fully awake and energetic as the topic moved to his reason for living...Tai Chi.

He had gained enough energy to take my wife and me out to lunch at one of his favorite restaurants, where we used to go many years ago after mornings of practice. The entire time he was animated as he talked about Tai Chi, old students, his son and family. At this point he told me of his desire to no longer live if he could no longer teach. It was his life, his focus, and if he couldn't work with students, he didn't want to go on living.

We bid each other goodbye after lunch, each wishing the other good luck in forming new classes. I had a strong feeling that I had said my final farewell, and felt sad under my happiness at having spent these precious hours with him. I wrote him once, sending a newspaper article about my winning the Push Hands Grand Championship at Taste of China, a prestigious Tai Chi tournament. A month or so later I received a letter from his son Frank, informing me of his death. He also said how happy Master Choy had been at my success. Sadness and loss mixed with happiness, and I felt in touch with the theory of Yin and Yang. Master Choy will be sorely missed.

Much of what I am sharing comes through Master Choy, less so with other teachers, and most from inspiration gleaned from thousands of hours playing with Tai Chi. There are a few important points or classic teachings that make Tai Chi unique. The simple, basic movements of the Yang Style Long Form are repeated many times throughout, with subtle or complex variations added. The short forms cut out the repeats. In this book you will encounter basic advice and practical information relayed in many variations.

I am especially intrigued by Push Hands in all its aspects, so you'll find lots of thoughts on that subject. When I was growing up, my friends and I used to play a game known as Indian wrestling, which is almost identical to Push Hands. So you might say I've been doing Push Hands most of my life. For some reason in the early years of my Tai Chi practice and teaching, I held back from playing Push Hands, thinking it too competitive for my peaceful state of mind. At some point I got interested, and now realize how much profound knowledge is contained in Push Hands. In fact I would venture to say that if you don't explore Push Hands, you'll never know Tai Chi Chuan as a complete art.

I also want to thank all the students I've worked with who have supported me in my exploration of this infinite topic. Their questions and problems cause me to look within, and try and come up with a way to help them discover from within, the essence of Tai Chi Chuan. Nothing brings me greater joy then to see that "Ah-Ha" come to someone. For me, like Master Choy, that is what makes life worth living. I sincerely hope that this little book will give you some "Ah-Ha's" and help you to find more enjoyment and satisfaction with your Tai Chi practice.

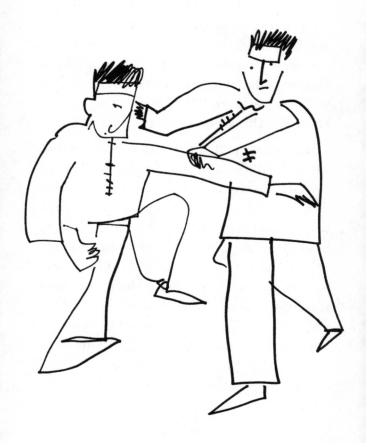

A String of Pearls

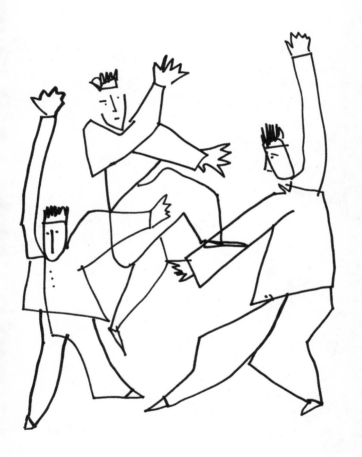

1 Approach your practice of Tai Chi with a mixture of awe, respect and love. Realize that people have been doing the same movements that you are now doing for at least twenty generations, and every time you start, the cumulative greatness of this art is expressed through you. You are the forward edge of a wave that is moving end-lessly forward, pushed by the entire ocean of past experience.

2 When emitting energy, think of a gun. The legs are the stock of the rifle, the arms the barrel. When you pull the trigger (Yi or mind is mobilized into action) there is an explosion which results in a release of energy. The stock (legs) take the recoil so the energy can be focused out the barrel. The barrel must be straight and pointed where you want the energy to go. You can imagine what would happen if your barrel was crooked. Make sure to line up your body, so that the power can move through smoothly.

3 Every part of the body is a hand and every part of the body is hooked up to the center. No part of the body can be touched without the whole being affected. Imagine a spider has spun a web that fills your body. The center of the web is your Dan Tien. The spider waits at the center with its eight arms attached to silk that connects the eight directions. Any little movement in any part of the web is transmitted to

the spider in the center. The spider can tell from experience what has gotten in its web and reacts accordingly. Through Push Hands practice, we learn when and how to deal with energy that moves into our energy field. But you must be patient while you wait for something to come your way. Nourish your internal spider by breathing into your Dan Tien.

4 The Alchemists of old spent most of their time trying to turn the base elements into gold. No one has yet accomplished that, as far as I know. The Taoists were alchemists of their bodies. They wanted to turn the base energies (Jieng and Chi) into the rarest of energies (Shen). I believe many have done that. So if you accomplish turning lead into gold you get rich. If you turn Jieng and Chi into Shen you gain immortality. You choose which is more worth the effort

5 There are 26 bones in each foot, 26 bones in each hand for a total of 104 bones just in the hands and feet. In the entire body there are 206 bones, so that means that over half of the bones of the body are in the hands and feet. Between each bone there is a joint which allows varying degrees of mobility. So when you practice Tai Chi be aware of the almost infinite variety of possible movements with the hands and feet. When playing Push Hands, use this incredible adaptability to respond to the slightest movement of your opponent.

6 The more one plays with Tai Chi, the more one's mind sees Tai Chi in everything. Someone was talking about a jazz instructor who had written on the board his philosophy for learning jazz. When I heard it, I couldn't help thinking that he was really talking about the best way to learn Tai Chi. On the board were written three words: imitate, assimilate, and innovate.

How true. Imitate your teacher and Masters; assimilate their teaching and movements and make them yours; innovate and help Tai Chi grow and change. Learn the classics, understand what they are, then move on. Respect the past, experience the present, and prepare for the future. So it turns out that Tai Chi and jazz have a great deal in common.

7 In Tai Chi practice, as in life in general, it is not what you do, but how you do it. Doing one movement correctly is much more beneficial then doing many movements incorrectly. Adhere to the classics, practice, have patience, and you will attain mastery. It is within all our grasps.

8 The practice of Tai Chi, and especially Push Hands, demonstrates the ability of the human body to react to a situation totally, without having to run the action

through the conscious mind. In the beginning, yes, we think about how we want to move and why. As our practice deepens and integrates into us at a cellular level, we use natural, reflexive movement. Practice until you reach that level and you will be experiencing a miracle.

9 The classic teachings of Tai Chi and Taoism are often obscured in trying to make much ado about nothing. Energy movement in the body follows natural laws of physics. There is nothing secret or mystical about reaching the highest levels in your Tai Chi practice. Observe the workings of the universe and align yourself with that. Use your will power and you will attain.

10 I watched a woman, five feet tall and 100 pounds Push Hands with a man who is six feet six and 260 pounds. At first, many people thought "how silly," yet

both learned a great deal. The woman was determined and pushed like a wild animal caught in a trap. She managed to throw him off balance more than once! The man had to become soft and play like a mother cat with her young. He had to use plenty of restraint to play on her level and still learn. Never turn down an opportunity to push with anybody. You'll always learn something.

11 The process of matching breath with movement is a step along the path to simple movement. It is an exercise and not an end point. When doing Tai Chi at an advanced level, there is no consideration of breath. The breathing should be natural, relaxed, and responsive to the demand placed on it. When playing Push Hands or doing sparring, your breath will of course be shorter and less full. One benefit of practicing Tai Chi is that the breath will be deeper and more relaxed no matter what the

demand, but don't let anyone tell you that you will not breathe quickly and perspire when exerting through the form, Push Hands, or sparring. Be realistic in the expectations placed on your body and mind.

12 The more powerful the imagination of how you want the energy to move in the body, the greater will be the actual result. When doing the form or Push Hands, visualize the energy interacting between your hands and the earth and back up again and you will be pleased with the results. Align your body so that the energy that moves down and back up can do so with very little in the way of restriction and resistance. You will be amazed at the results.

13 Hopefully we can arrive at a place in our study of Tai Chi where we can practice with what I call "advanced beginner's mind." That means that we gaze upon the form as fresh and new each time we start to move. We have arrived at a place where we don't have to think about what movement comes next or how to do it. That part has been mastered. Then it is possible just to be amazed at what the body is doing and how it feels at each moment. It is like exploring random movement, yet the body is moving according to the deep cellular learning that has gone before. Beginner's mind is possible at the start of your learning when you truly are a beginner or anytime when practicing with a teacher (for then you don't have to think or move on your own). "Advanced beginners mind" happens after mastering the form.

14 The body is most efficient when the spine is erect, the chest and shoulders are relaxed, and all parts are as close to the center of gravity as is practical. One of the secrets of good Push Hands play is to gently lead the opponent into leaning and moving his parts away from the center. Do this gradually and with extreme softness, and the opponent will never know until it is too late. If you threaten, he will be reluctant to come out after you.

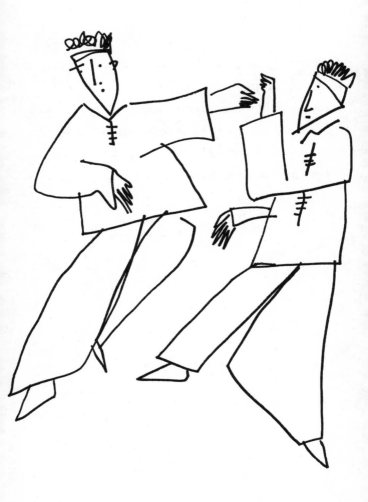

15 Having a good teacher is so very important in learning Tai Chi. Books and videos can help, but offer no feedback. Respect your teacher and observe the rules. If you don't feel you can do this, find another teacher.

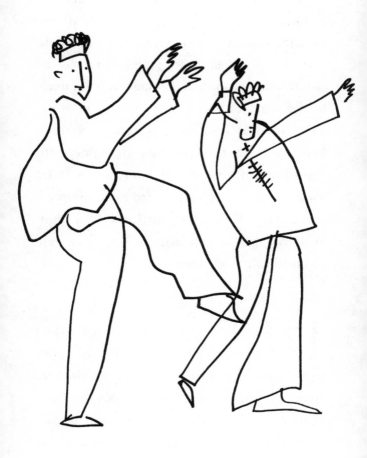

16 Any emotional stress will affect the physical body. If you think fear, for instance, your body will go through all the psychophysical changes to prepare you to deal with this perceived stress. If this stress is not relieved, much damage can be done to the muscles and cells of your body. It is like pressure building up behind a dam. You must let this pressure dissipate, and your Tai Chi form is a wonderful way to let some of the stress release from the muscles and organs. If you do your form on a regular basis, the tension will not have a chance to build to a high level.

17 Rituals evolve from need. If a farmer needs water and he does something that results in water, the chances are good that he will repeat the same action again. If a baseball player is on a streak, many times he will continue to do any and all behaviors he has been doing in order to keep his luck going. Tai Chi evolved from ritualistic dance like movements that brought improved health, happiness, and martial skill. These movements worked so they were expanded and repeated. When you practice your form, you are hooking up to energy that reaches back thousands of years. These movements have been handed from person to person. It is almost as if you could touch with your own hands the very first person who ever did Tai Chi like movements. He or she might have been doing these movements for the very same reasons that you are. Don't forget to give your respect to your ancestors.

18 Your life should flow out of your Tai Chi practice. There is a state when your practice and your life become one and you are always practicing Tai Chi, aware of each moment completely.

19 Our Tai Chi training moves from large to small. When we start our studies of Tai Chi, our forms should be larg-

er than they will end up being. It is like carving a figure out of stone. You must work your way in toward the finished product slowly. If you go too far, there is no turning back. Your Tai Chi form will naturally get smaller as you gain control of energy. We want to do the most with the least if we want to conserve energy. You can usually tell at what point a student studied with a teacher by how large the student's form is. The early students of Yang Chen Fu, for instance, learned the form when Master Yang was doing a larger frame form. As he got older and his form naturally got smaller, the students who started at that point would think that their form was the only way. It is very difficult for a young, strong student to start studying with a teacher who is at the end of his or her career or life. The teacher must be very good to encourage the student to start out larger then the teacher is currently moving. If an older teacher just encourages imitation of movement, there will be trouble for the student as he develops.

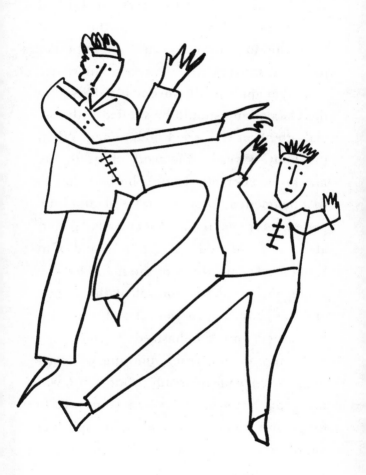

20 Have patience. It usually takes many years just to learn the Tai Chi movements and principles, and the rest of your life to improve. You start with the physical movements, learning the basic rules that apply to all movements. These are the classics and should be studied with special attention to correct body usage. When the body is ready, the work shifts to the mental or energetic level. The body has to first be opened, loosened, relaxed, and integrated before energy is concentrated, generated, and focused. Meditation and Chi Kung are the practices of the mental stage. When the mind has control of the energy and the body is open and relaxed, the spiritual aspects are emphasized. If your body and mind are not ready, nothing will happen. When you are ready, your spirit will move on its own. It is then your task to focus and channel this Shen or spiritual energy and you attain the ultimate goal of self realization.

21 Relaxation is a key to successful Tai Chi practice. Yet you must be sure to relax with full attention. This relaxation is like a full balloon, not an empty one. It is like a rock delicately balanced on the top of a mountain, not sitting on flat ground. It is standing balanced on two feet with head held high, not lying down flat. It is the state of dynamic equilibrium, of potential, of possibilities.

22 Internal energy is known as bone energy, as opposed to muscle energy. If you want to use internal energy, line up your bones. Keep in mind that between each bone and its neighbor is a joint. For maximum use of body dynamics and internal power, limit bending at the joints. The elbow is the connecting joint for the upper arm and lower arm. The more you bend this joint, the more responsibility is placed on the connecting tissues. The same is true with the wrist. Make sure to line up the lower part of the palm (you can feel the forearm bones) with the object to be pushed. If you try and push with the upper palm or fingers, the connective tissue of the hand will have to deal with the stress. It is very easy to pull the fingers back and hold them back. A little study of how the body is constructed goes a long way.

23 Don't be afraid of habits. They allow us to relax. Habits can prepare us for what is to come. When I get up in the morning to practice Tai Chi, I have a specific sequence that I go through. As soon as I get to my practice place, my mind and body know what is going to happen and I am already entering a state of relaxation. When I start to move in the form, my mind and body do not have to think or wonder about what is going to happen. Every cell of my being has been through Tai Chi and knows how to do it's job. There is no arguing between my cells about who will get to do what. It is a well organized team; having been trained together, they are able to communicate on a deep level. Acting without thinking is enlightenment. Habits gained through training are helpful.

24 It is said that the present players of Tai Chi do not even remotely approach the skill level of the masters of old. I disagree. The seeds have been planted in us. With the proper mixture of fire (will power), earth (dedication), air (inspiration), and water (correct teaching), we can attain the ultimate end of Tai Chi—reaching harmony with the Tao. I don't think it is important to be able to throw an opponent across the room with a touch. The enlightened nature is expressed as sensitive, loving, caring, peaceful, and understanding so that there are no opponents to throw. Keep the energy gained by practice moving toward those goals and you'll enjoy life to the fullest.

25 Most people pay much more attention to what they wear than what their bones and muscles are doing, until there is some problem. Tai Chi is the study of the body as it moves through space. What could possibly be more interesting and rewarding?

26 Reaction time covers three phases: time required 1) to sense the signal, 2) to decide on the correct response, and 3) to respond. The greatest aid to quick response is training. We detect stimuli with our senses, and in descending order of speed they are sight, sound, touch, smell, and taste. In the fastest group (sight) there is another factor that comes into play. A signal appearing from above (overhead) will provide a quicker response then one arriving from below. So for fighting and Push Hands, fake from above and deliver energy from below.

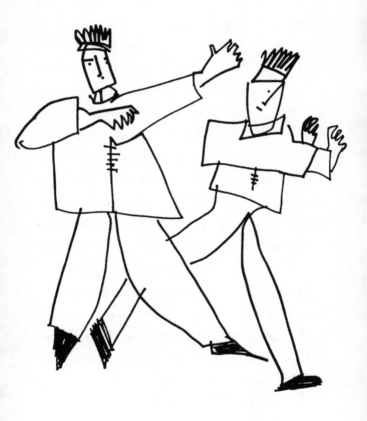

27 The concept of Wu Chi to Tai Chi is paramount to understanding Taoism and Tai Chi Chuan. Wu Chi is the state of complete balance, nothing and everything, the all inclusive void. At some point the balance is shifted so that Yin and Yang are formed. In perfect balance Yin and Yang combine, and only through imbalance do they appear. Our lives contain two movements. The first is the movement from nothing (birth) to something (maturity). This is a Yang phase of life, the movement outward and upward. At the peak of our maturity, the Yin phase starts. We start our movement back down and in toward Wu Chi and reuniting with the Tao. It is the natural way of the universe, and man is a part of nature. Observe nature and you can understand how things can be and are. Our Tai Chi form is a ritualistic dance that plays out this process. We start by standing in perfect balance Wu Chi. At some point a thought comes to us to set us into imbalance and then starts the movement back and forth from Yin to Yang and Yang to Yin

until, at some point we return to balance
and Wu Chi. This is a wonderful opportunity to observe the birth of energy, experience the fullness of each moment, and
prepare for death. Wu Chi to Tai Chi—
Tai Chi to Wu Chi.

28 The form is not Tai Chi. It is but a
tool to do something else. It is like
using a computer. We do not use computers
just to sit and punch keys. We use the computer to do something, to help us accomplish a goal. The form is like the computer
in that we don't do the form just to do the
form, but use the form to practice moving
energy inside our body, gain powers of con-
centration, learn relaxation, build internal
and external strength, and experience psychophysical integration. I urge students to
look beyond the form to the true purpose of
the study of Tai Chi Chuan.

29 One of the best exercises to increase your awareness of each movement in your Tai Chi form is to break it down, one movement at a time and explore all the possibilities to that movement. Do it slow and fast, low stance or high. Add Fa Jing, change the breathing pattern, and most importantly, do it as big as you can and really let go into the essential nature of how the limbs are tied to the center. From big, work your way to very small and still be aware of the movement in the center. Find the smallest possible movement at the center, and work your way back to large. Notice how the limbs get activated as the movement grows. Feel free to dissect each and every minute part of each movement and play with it. Don't get too serious or the movements will not flow. After all, Tai Chi is body movement directed by the mind. Think about Buddha sitting or reclining with that lovely smile on his face. He knew that the answer to life was a smile. You'll go a long way if you can smile when doing your form or playing Push Hands.

30 If you have a thought in your head:

> *you cannot see*
> *you cannot hear*
> *you cannot taste*
> *you cannot feel*
> *you cannot think.*

In order to do any of these things completely, the mind needs to be quiet and
still, open and receptive. Thoughts block
reality because they are of the past. By the
time they have reached the place where
you can hear them in your head, they are
past. We can, of course, do many things at
one time, yet we are not fully present if
thoughts are also present. Practice Tai Chi
until the thinking mind disappears into
the movement.

31 Ever since the earliest of times,
man has done ritualized dance to
win the favor of the gods. The dance served
the purpose of strengthening the spirit of
the warriors, bringing the community

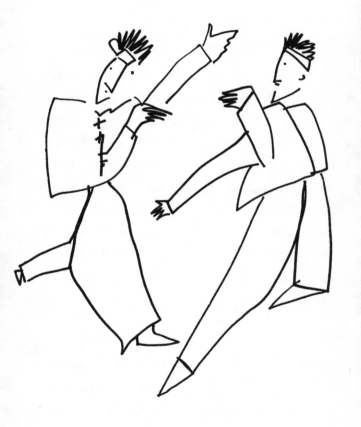

together for common purpose, winning the favor of the opposite sex, and blending with the intention of the gods. Tai Chi did and does accomplish these goals.

32 Make sure you line up the body so you can push with the legs and trunk of your body. Any angle or bend results in a loss of energy and effectiveness. It is especially important that the angle of the shoulder never exceed 180°, or straight out to the sides. Be careful not to let the elbows get behind the body which opens the shoulder joints too much. If the shoulder opens beyond 180° and the arm gets behind the body, the muscles and connective tissue will have to bear the load instead of the bones. Actually, having the arms as straight as possible without being locked and as close to the body as possible without pressing tightly against the side is even better. Imagine pushing a heavy load with a stick in front of you. If the stick is straight, you can get your body behind it and not lose much strength. But put an angle in the stick and you will see that there is a great loss in power. The joint or bend will have to deal with the force. It is quite simple.

33 It is a fact that every action of our body requires energy. Our basic metabolic rate is the base amount of energy our bodies require to exist. When we do work, a chemical reaction occurs using stored energy and leaving behind waste products. It is like burning a log in a fire. We end up with ash and heat. Or burning gas in an automobile leaves carbon monoxide and many other chemicals. There is nothing yet discovered that will use energy and not leave some waste. Our bodies are the same. We use energy and have waste to deal with. If the chemical residue is not eliminated, the results range from a dull ache to complete shut down of the system. Rest allows the body to move the toxins out. Tai Chi is designed to allow for periods of rest following periods of work, and usually half of the body works while the other half rests. There are also two very important periods of rest that I call the top and bottom of a roller coaster ride. It is the moment when up changes to down or down changes to up. When Yin changes to Yang and Yang to Yin. It is the moment between inhale and exhale. It is the crack in the wall to the infinite, it is the moment of enlightenment. Seek this moment out and gently stretch it with awareness. Your body and mind will find renewal.

34 Enlightenment is most often experienced at a moment that occurs between the in breath and out breath. This special place is like a small crack in the cosmic egg. If we look close enough through this crack, we can glimpse the true workings of the universal energy or Tao. It is the goal of Tai Chi and most meditative arts to expand this moment, stretch this tear in the fabric that clouds our vision, allow relaxation, clear the mind so we can have this experience. Tai Chi is done very slowly, the breath is allowed to deepen and slow, the body is relaxed and strengthened, a firm is root established, all so that our super conscious or higher self can reunite with the Tao. Enlightenment is not an all or nothing, now or never experience. It is more like walking out a door into a new place. As we open the door we get a glimpse of what is on the other side. The wider the door, the more we see. The further out of the door way, the more we can see until we finally close the door and are completely in this new place and this is our reality. The old place is only a memory, a dream. We are now in a place where we can really be of assistance to others, to help make the planet a more comfortable place for all in existence.

35 Try an experiment. Stand up straight and without bending your knees see how high you can jump. Now squat down and see how high you can jump. Next, take a little hop and jump. I'm sure you can see that the greater the compression of your energy, the greater the resulting release. In Tai Chi, we compress our own energy by shifting the weight onto squatting legs, use a partner to help us by doing Push Hands, or practice Chi Kung exercises to compress and focus energy with breath and mind. We can channel this energy and use it for growth, healing, and enlightenment. Blocks in the tissues, joints, organs, or meridians can be opened. The gates on the microcosmic and macrocosmic orbit can be opened. The chakras can be energized. These are all positive results of the mind directing the energy. Now think about what happens if you don't release the build up of compressive type energy that results from stress, fear, and anxiety. High blood pressure, strokes, heart attacks, chronic fatigue, back problems and so many more are symptoms of a build up of internal pressure that hasn't been dealt with. Practice Tai Chi and the energy will be moved, smoothed, and grounded. Just do your form and relax.

36 Push Hands should more correctly be called "Moving Bodies." The hands are actually a small part of the actual act of moving someone off balance. The hands are mostly for delivering information to the brain about the opponent's movement. Most of the pushing is done with the trunk and legs.

37 One of the many wonderful things about Tai Chi is that it can be practiced anywhere and at anytime. The slow, relaxed movements allow a feeling of harmonizing with the surrounding environment. Some times I play with my Tai Chi practice by allowing the environment to shape my movements. When practicing by the ocean, I feel the rhythm and power of the waves push me forward. The stillness and heat of the desert melts me into my center. On the top of a mountain I can feel the root and support allow me to truly lift my spirit upward. The swiftness of a rushing river, the intensity of a city park, the familiarity of my backyard all affect and help my Tai Chi practice become more than just exercise.

38 The arms and legs are what is known as appendages of the trunk (spine and pelvis). Our earliest ancestors (fish) didn't have well developed appendages. The trunk was used to move about. If you watch a fish move you will notice that a small movement at its center will result in a quick movement forward. One of the most powerful ways to improve your Tai Chi movement, either in form or Push Hands, is to think of yourself as a fish with very limited use of hands and legs. Just move your center and watch what happens.

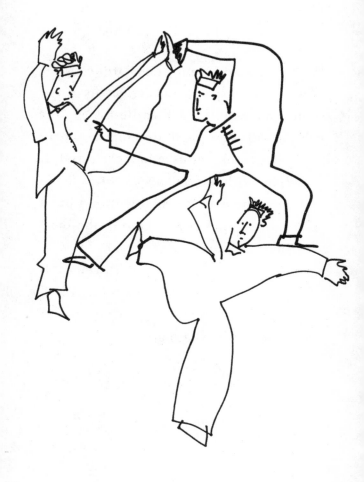

39 Running water clears itself. Keep the energy rivers of your body moving and they will balance and clear out toxins.

40 Yi is the mind or intention. Every action is preceded by an intention. If our opponent wants to push us, first his mind will make the decision. If we are sensitive enough, we can feel this impulse or brain wave form. You must pay attention. The Yi then sends the signal to the body and the Chi starts to build. The Chi moves the muscles, so it must build to a certain level before there is movement. If you are sensitive enough you can feel this build up. Finally, the body moves and this is expressed as Jing. This we all feel, yet if we listen carefully, we can control this release before it is too strong. So the highest level of Push Hands training is to listen to the opponent's mind, then feel the Chi build before there is movement, then finally deal in a relaxed fashion with the Jing.

41 A law of physics states that a body in motion tends to remain in motion in a straight line. In Tai Chi Push Hands we turn our body to neutralize the incoming push which will then go straight by us. For the same reason it is very important that we have a good, solid brake for our forward movement by rooting our front foot before we move onto it. If you step and push at the same time, it is easy to get thrown off balance. So the process always is to step a foot out without moving the trunk, then move the weight onto it.

42 Gravity is always pulling the mass of the body downward. When we take one part of the body away from the center of gravity, it should be balanced by an opposing part. As you study the Tai Chi forms you'll notice this is always true. Think about trying to carry a heavy weight on one side. It is much easier to balance the load by carrying equal loads on both sides (like a yoke), or right on the center (like a bundle on top of the head).

43 There are three basic foot positions in the martial arts. For close in arts like Judo and Aikido, the feet are fairly close together to allow very quick movement in any direction. For long distance arts like Karate and Tae Kwan Do, the stance is quite wide to provide a solid base for strong kicks and punches. Because of the distance to the opponent, movements don't have to be as quick. Mid-range arts like Tai Chi and Hsing Yi use an intermediate stance which is a compromise between the quickness of a narrow stance and the power of a wide stance.

44 Double weighted is having deep roots on both feet at the same time. Relaxation can happen in this posture, but not movement. For quick movement, the body has to be right on the edge of unbalance while still being balanced. In Tai Chi Classic teachings this is known as a fly cannot land on us without setting us in motion. Watch an animal while it is hunting. It is always in a state of readiness, just on the edge. Stand on a Teeter Totter (a plank balanced on log) and find a balance by placing one foot on either side of the center. If you shift your weight even a tiny bit, you'll easily upset the balance. Our reactions must be quick and correct in order to make minute adjustments. In Tai Chi form and Push Hands, we are always like that. There is no time when we get off this Teeter Totter.

45 It is a physical law that any action is met by a reaction that is always equal and opposite. If you press on a spring, your force is met with an equal force coming back at you. This law may not always be evident because different materials (air, water, solids) react in different ways. In our bodies, a pressure will result in a compression of our cells, and when the pressure is released, the cells will spring back to the original shape. A pull causes the cells to separate, and when released, will also spring back. In Tai Chi Classic teaching, we call this borrowing energy. The opponent pushes me which compresses my cells, causing my energy to compress against the floor. The energy builds up against the floor, and when the push stops, either by my opponent withdrawing, or my warding off this energy, the compression is released in the opposite direction which means back to him. The Tai Chi form is constant practice on how to compress energy and direct its release.

46 Reflexes are nature's most perfect self defense device. The stimuli does not have to be processed by the conscious mind (Yi). The body reacts much more quickly than if our mind tried to instruct the body to move. In Tai Chi we want to train the reflexes to act and to remove the conscious mind. Then you will have true speed.

47 The crouch is a powerful position. Think of a tiger about to spring, or a horse about to jump. This gathering of energy into the front of the hip is what is known as using your Kua. In order to "borrow" your opponent's energy, you allow him to move his energy into your Kua by pushing you into a crouch, then, at the proper moment, release it back into him.

48 Man's posture is mostly determined by how he thinks he should look and move. We are conditioned to stand and move in ways that we have been taught from the outside, and these are mostly determined by society. Think of the posture of a soldier, a model, a loser. We can pick out these people just by how they stand and move. An actor can come on stage, and without a word, we can know a great deal about what that person will do and how they will act. The goal of Tai Chi practice is to form feelings from the inside out so as to harmonize and balance our body. We move from thinking to feeling, from outside in to inside out. Instead of causing situations, we react to them. Instead of pushing, we join and flow with the energy.

49 Moving in Tai Chi is like walking across a swift moving stream. Your foot has to be well rooted before you shift your weight onto it. Try walking in a river sometime and see what happens if you don't root first. You'll be swept downstream.

50 We have three major storage vessels for energy in the body: the lower, middle, and upper Dan Tien. It is very important to fill the lower reservoir first, then the middle, and finally the top. It will be a waste of effort to try and fill the top first as the energy will flow to the bottom, as is natural. There are people that try and fill the top without first filling the bottom by the use of special exercises or drugs. In the long run that always leads to disaster as there is no ground to deal with the increase in energy. You need a solid foundation if you are going to explore the outermost reaches of your psyche. So take your time and work from the bottom up. Learn to root and ground your energy, relax your body and mind and consciously control internal energy. Do standing meditations, breathe into your lower Dan Tien until you can feel energy there, then work your way up. You will not regret the time spent in preparation.

51 The dragon is a wonderful beast. Its long tail can drag on the ground behind and offer support. Imagine you have a long, solid tail that comes straight down from the end of your spine and hits the ground. When doing your form, rely on the support the tail provides. Another image to help with balance is the tripod. Because it has three points for balance, it can be very stable on all types of terrain. Imagine you have another leg that comes down from your spine and use it for support.

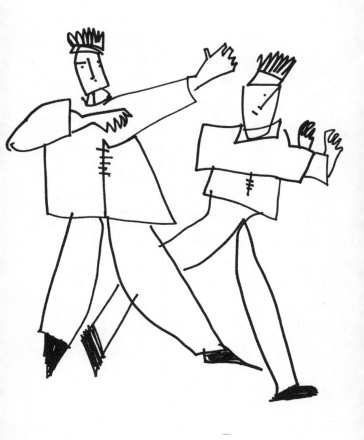

52 The process of learning Tai Chi requires patience. Slow and steady progress comes with regular practice. This should be augmented with occasional retreats or intensive workshops to push you to a new level. Also be careful not to compare your progress with others. Hopefully, the journey to mastery of Tai Chi brings joy all along the path.

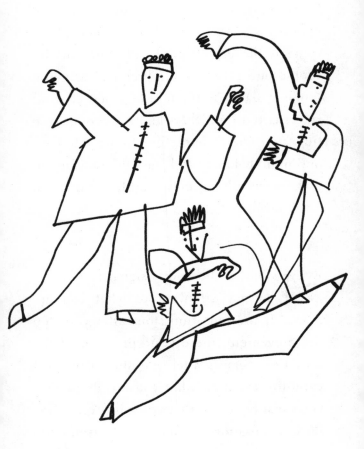

49

53 The body's structure resembles a tent with a center pole that is held in an upright position by guy wires that oppose each other resulting in balance. Your spine is the center pole and your muscles should pull evenly in all directions to maintain easy balance. If one side (front, back, or sides) is too tight there must be compensation somewhere. Therefore, in order to have optimum balance and ease of movement, make sure all muscles maintain an equal level of tone.

54 Pain is the body's signal to tell you to pay attention to what you are doing. If the sensation stops after you stop the movement, there is no problem. If the sensation persists after you stop, you must carefully examine what you are doing. Yet you must be aware that you will experience muscle sensations as you train yourself to do movements you haven't done before. The usual sensation is a dull ache. This is common in all athletics. But if you experience a

sharp, shooting sensation you should immediately stop and examine what you are doing
for any incorrect movement. Do not continue if shooting sensations persist.

55 Always prepare your muscles for the
load. You could probably stop a car
from rolling down a hill if you are attached
and have your muscles ready before you let
the brake off. If you take the brake off
before you get prepared, the result will not
be good. In Push Hands, you can not wait
for your opponent's force to gather momentum before you try and deal with it. Attach
yourself to the energy as far away from your
center as you can while still maintaining
your center of balance. This is the principle
of listening and neutralizing.

56 Strength and power aren't the same
thing. Strength is the ability to do
work. Force times distance equals strength.
To lift one hundred pounds one foot doesn't

take as much strength as it does to lift fifty pounds five feet. Strength does not consider time. Power is strength divided by time. In the martial arts we are concerned with power, not strength. Who can deliver the most energy in the shortest time. The three elements that are important in fighting are, in order of importance, speed, power, and technique. In Tai Chi, we want to think that isn't true, that technique is the most important. Push Hands is a special game that is part of the Tai Chi training for fighting. Push Hands still trains speed in reactions, power in pushes, and various techniques, yet relies less on speed then does fighting.

57 The body is composed of trillions of cells, all individuals, that can repair and reproduce themselves to varying degrees. It is the unconscious mind (Hsin) and the conscious mind (Yi) that organize and direct. The practice of Tai Chi helps the Hsin and Yi to work together and focus the energy of the super-conscious or universal mind.

58 There is a natural law that states that form follows function. The body develops to deal with situations and stresses placed upon it. If the body is required to do heavy work, it develops large muscles. If one draws a great deal, the small motor muscles of the hands get developed. When one practices Tai Chi many hours a day, the whole body learns to move as one unit. The muscles are toned without much increase in bulk. The bones get strong as well as flexible. You can almost always pick out a Tai Chi player by his or her body.

59 The classics teach us to "Seek stillness in movement." If you think about a wheel turning, you will notice that as the outside of the wheel turns a great distance, the hub turns very little. When you play Tai Chi, your Yi or conscious mind is like the hub and remains calm, quiet, and relaxed as the rest of the body moves. If your Yi is placed on the Dan Tien when doing solo practice, there will be a sense of attentive stillness when moving. When working with a partner, let your Yi be like a mirror that faces your partner reflecting and matching his movements without thought. Or imagine your Yi to be like water that surrounds, engulfs, reacts with, yields to, and never separates from your partner's energy. If you play in the water, you will notice that as you move your hand, say on a horizontal plane, the water sticks to the front, flows smoothly around, and fills in immediately behind arm as it cuts through. There are no vacant spaces. So when playing Push Hands, let your body be like that water and stick to your opponent without tension. This is only truly possible if your mind is centered and calm with your body relaxed and yet full of attention. It takes much dedicated practice to arrive at that level, so get to work and don't waste your time.

60 Imagine you are enclosed in a large bubble that extends about one-and-a-half feet beyond your body. When you do your form or do Push Hands, work at the edge of this bubble. Don't let your opponent inside. Think of it as your castle. Once outside your castle you are quite vulnerable. When playing Push Hands, make sure you have good reason to move your troops outside the castle. Also, be very careful when letting your opponent inside. The area of relative safety (the edge of your bubble) is quite small.

61 The knees are the most stressed joint in the body when playing Tai Chi. Many people who practice Tai Chi experience knee problems, so to limit the possibility of doing any harm to your knees, follow these simple rules. The knee always moves in the direction the toe is headed. Be careful not to let the knee collapse inward when moving onto it. When sitting on the rear leg, be sure to still keep the knee headed in the direction the rear toe is headed. The knee just covers the toe when moving forward. If you move so that the knee extends past the toe you will place a great burden on the knee joint. If you do not

cover the toe with the knee you will not be getting maximum exercise. Never lock the knee. The knee always maintains a very slight bend when straightened. Try not to let the knee move in a lateral direction when doing any movement. Be careful, practice with mindfulness, and your knees will end up being strengthened and opened.

62 In order to do the Tai Chi Chuan solo form, you must realize that each movement is a real movement, like a punch, kick or block, that is pantomimed and done slowly. These are fast self defense movements that are done slowly in order to understand them in great detail, figure out the alignment of body and Chi, coordinate breath, and relax. If you do not understand what you are doing in a martial sense, you can't possibly do Tai Chi Chuan. There are many people, even teachers, that object to thinking about the martial side of Tai Chi. I'm sure that without a martial understanding, a person will never master this art.

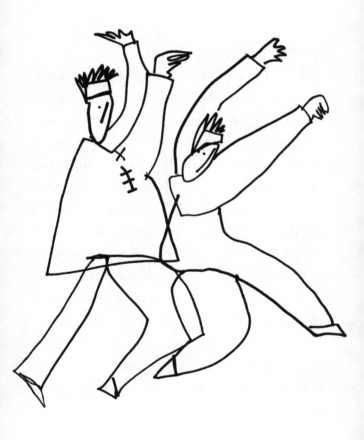

63 The average body uses about 85% of its available energy just to exist, breathe, move the blood, digest the food, and keep the glands working. That leaves only 15% for other activities. In times of stress we borrow from this base amount and as a result our normal functions are shut down for a while. It then takes time to regain this 85% so everything return to normal. In Tai Chi we learn how to do the most with the least so we don't have to steal energy from our 85%. The experienced Tai Chi player probably uses less than 85% anyway as his or her body is more relaxed, breathes deeper and less frequently, and has a great ability to control most of the energy movement in the body.

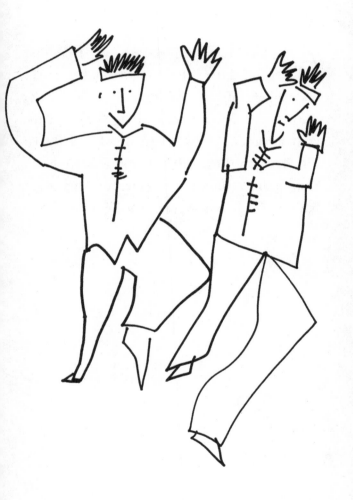

64 Develop your particular strengths and skills. There is no need to work on aspects of yourself that don't respond well. If you are big and strong, use that to your advantage. If you are small and flexible, develop those skills. If you want to be a champion, exploit the unique body that you have. A snake will never be a tiger.

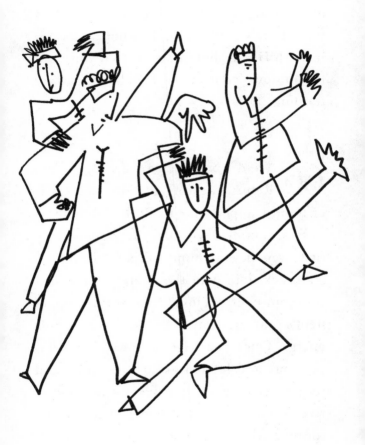

65 If you want to train your performance power, you must train your muscles at a speed equal to or greater then that of the event. Strength is not important in Push Hands, but power is, so if you want to improve your Push Hands, do power training.

66 Yield (Neutralize), Lead, Relax, Return the Energy. This process is of utmost importance in Push Hands practice. Always deal with the incoming energy first even if your mind has already started an attack. Join with the energy and lead it into your center (close) to borrow the opponent's energy. Don't try to redirect this energy. Once you have borrowed the energy, relax and let it sink to your spine and root. Only then will you be in a position to release and return the energy back to the source. All this happens in an instant, almost simultaneously.

67 Our body is like a spring fed lake. The lake gets Yang Chi from the heavens in the form of rain, and Yin Chi from the earth in the form of an underground spring. They mix to form the lake. Our bodies get heavenly or Yang Chi through the Bai Hui point on the top of the head. The Yin Chi rises from the earth and is absorbed by our body through the Yung Chuan point on the bottom of the foot. These are mixed, balanced, and stored in our Dan Tien. If the pond gets too much rain or the spring is too active, there is a flood. If there is no rain or the spring dries up, there is drought. The body is the same. We can tolerate either extreme for only a short time before the system is damaged beyond repair. If the body is getting too full, we need to drain off or divert the excess. Conversely, if there isn't enough energy coming in from the usual sources, we need to find another source. The practice of Tai Chi is designed to open the Bai Hui and Yung Chuan so that Yin and Yang Chi can move freely in, out, and around so that balance can easily be attained

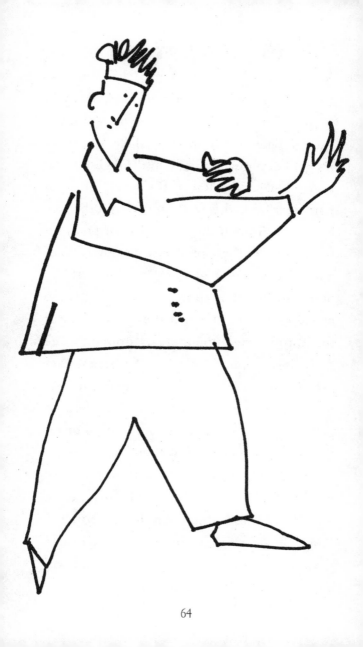

68 Before starting your practice, be sure to take a moment to hook up your basic energy points to your Dan Tien. To do this you concentrate your mind first on your Dan Tien, then on the Yung Chuan points on the bottoms of the feet, the Bai Hui on the top of the head, and the Lao Kung in the center of the palms. Since energy follows the mind, these points will be strung together, like a string of pearls, just by concentrating on them. The deeper your attention to these points, the stronger the connection will be.

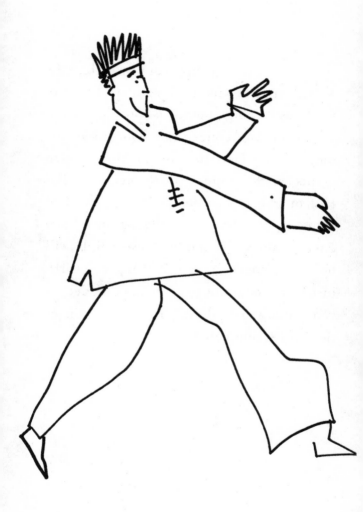

69 I am always suspicious of someone who claims to be a healer. There is no such thing as a "healer." The universe is the only thing that can heal. Some people can interact with energy in a way that can help others to use the universal energy to enhance their own healing. It is similar to saying "I am enlightened." If one was enlightened there would be no separate "I" to say so. The ego will limit one's ability to become one with the universe, so be careful.

70 Man is probably the only creature on earth that forms habits that are detrimental to his health and the smooth functioning of his body. Society has caused more damage then nature ever has. Just look at tight clothes that restrict movement, high heel shoes that tip the pelvis, chairs that hurt the back and shorten the hamstrings, cigarettes that restrict our breathing. When we practice Tai Chi we form a bond with our bodies that allows us to move beyond the limits of destructive habits into the open space of joyful and conscious movement.

71 Tai Chi Chuan and Chi Kung are very beneficial for controlling blood pressure. Think about the extremities (fingers, toes, top of head, base of spine) as openings for collecting or dispelling Chi. For high blood pressure, you want to move your energy downward and outward, and the reverse (inward and upward) for low blood pressure.

72 Energy makes itself available to us because we have a need for it. If we are already full, we will not receive more. When we are afraid, energy comes in order to deal with the situation. Anger also brings energy. So does laughter, happiness, and love. All make us more open to energy. Think about the times you were in love and I'm sure you will realize that you had almost unlimited energy. All of this emotional energy needs to be used or it can cause a problem of excess. Even love if not released can cause heart problems, high blood pressure, frustration, ulcers and the like. So be sure you let the emotional energy move through your body, and you'll really be available to receive more while giving more.

73 We have two large cavities in the body: the thoracic and the abdominal. The thoracic contains the lungs and heart. The movement of the diaphragm and

ribs cause gas (air) to enter and leave the lungs. There is an opening to the outside (nose and mouth) to allow this to happen and to make sure that there is not too great a build up of gas in the lungs. There is really no way to accumulate energy in this part of the body as any excess gas will always leave the body. The abdominal cavity is sealed to the outside. It is fluid filled (mostly water). It is for this reason that Tai Chi players emphasize abdominal breathing. If you add chi (heat) to this sealed area filled mostly with water, the fluid expands and gives off warmth which we can easily experience. The more energy which we direct to the lower belly (Dan Tien), the more energetic this fluid becomes. One of the properties of water is that it can hold energy (heat) for a long time. So when we practice Tai Chi and direct our energy to the Dan Tien, we store energy in this area that we can tap into for future use. Doing Tai Chi keeps the pot boiling on the stove!

74 Response must be adequate to meet the situation. For every stimulus there is a motor response. Tai Chi players learn how to limit the response to the minimum needed to meet the stimulus so as not to waste energy.

75 Every body is different with different roots and different branches. Each teacher or Master feels that what he or she is doing is right because it works for them. Listen to what each has to say, try it out if it makes sense to you, then add what feels right and reject what doesn't. Trust your intuition and your own body and develop your uniqueness.

76 The body needs to be in a state of perfect balance for Commencement of Tai Chi Chuan. Relaxed awareness that permeates every cell. Yin and Yang balanced. At this point not even a fly could land on the body without setting it into

motion. This balance is like a scale. When you add to one side, the other reacts. So let your Yi, or conscious mind be the fly that tips the scale and sends you into motion.

77 A good breathing meditation: stand straight and relax. Imagine that you are comfortably surrounded by a close fitting vacuum tube. When you inhale, your feet and head are gently pulled in opposite directions. When you exhale, there is a release. When you do this you will notice that as you inhale and lengthen, your belly will naturally pull inward, and as you relax back to center, your belly will naturally expand. This is known as prebirth breathing. Play with it and also try doing the opposite—when inhaling relax to center, and when exhaling, gently feel a pull in opposite directions. This is known as post birth breathing. See which feels more natural to you. Don't force your breath. As you relax, your breath will naturally get slower and deeper.

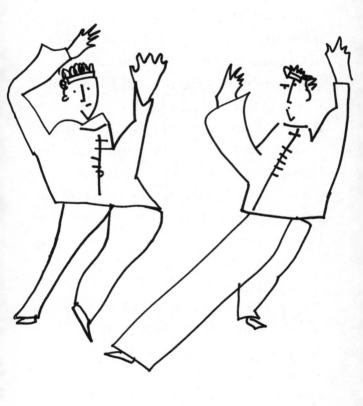

78 Moving energy in the body is enhanced by the use of the mind. Energy follows the mind so the more active your mind in the process of energy movement, the greater the results will be. Think of Chi as a basketball. If you just let the ball drop from waist height, it will bounce up a foot or two. If you throw it down with force, it will bounce much higher. Your internal energy is no different. Use your imagination to bounce your Chi from the floor to your hands. As the mind gains the power to concentrate, your Chi will increase and become more lively.

79 The Shen and Chi must be strengthened. You must think of yourself like a balloon or a tire. You need to be filled with spirit and energy in order to move smoothly. Then the push from the opponent can easily be redirected.

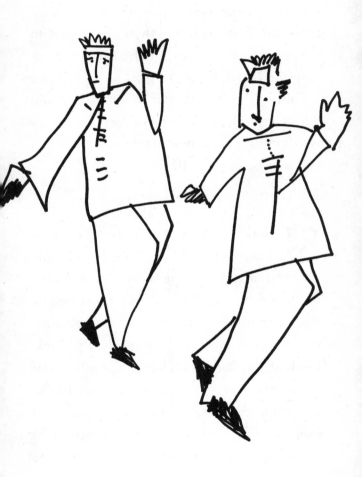

80 Yi, Chi, and Jing are very important concepts in Tai Chi Chuan. The mind (Yi) conceives of something, the energy of the body (Chi) is then channeled to accomplish this task, and finally the muscles and bones move (Jing). The greater the intention (Yi), the greater the internal build up (Chi), the greater the expression or result (Jing). So concentrate your mind and you will be happy with the results.

81 I don't think that it is a virtue to continue to do the form in the same way year after year. The form is ever changing and evolving. If you do the form exactly like your teacher after a few years of practice on your own, you are probably stuck. Look at any good teacher and notice how his or her form is different from day to day and moment to moment. The form is an expression of exactly where we are right now. Open up and allow inspiration to enter.

82 We must learn to distinguish between the opposites—Yin and Yang, substantial and insubstantial, hard and soft—so that energy will move. We need the two poles or Yin and Yang for life to exist. The Tai Chi player, in order to reach the highest levels, must be able to express these qualities when needed. That is enlightenment, knowing what to do when and being able to do it. Many players are afraid of expressing the Yang, or firm, in the belief that Tai Chi is only a soft and yielding martial art and practice. In the classics and history of Tai Chi, we often read about the Masters throwing opponents across the room. That sort of energy must be firm to support moving weight. When done correctly, it can be hard like a bat hitting a ball, or a wave crashing against the shore. Learn to do the most with what you have been given for a body, develop your strengths (sensitivity, flexibility, technique, internal energy, as well as muscle power) and you will be fulfilling your destiny.

83 The body is only as strong as its weakest part (usually a joint). Tai Chi is designed to strengthen unify and integrate all parts within the whole. You must develop your entire body with equal attention. If you play Push Hands, your partner will always seek out your weak part and keep at it until you figure out how to compensate for this weakness.

84 If you can visualize your skeleton doing Tai Chi, your form will be correct. Also, if you can visualize your partner's skeleton when playing Push Hands, you will be very effective by pushing his or her skeleton, not the surface. For healing, send energy into the bones to stimulate bone marrow production. In order to help your visualizations, get a good book on anatomy and physiology. That is important for any serious Tai Chi player.

85 Pay special attention to the joints. This is where the energy transfers from one part of the body to the next. It is easy to cut off or restrict energy at these junctures. Practice Silk Reeling to open the joints. Study the body very carefully in all the Tai Chi postures to make sure the energy has the shortest possible distance from root to branch (usually foot to hand). It is much like a hose in that any chink in the hose restricts the flow of water. If you feel pain in a part of the body while or after practicing Tai Chi, you most probably are blocking the flow of energy and it is accumulating somewhere. Look at yourself and try and feel exactly what is happening. Ask your teacher for help. He or she is trained to see these blocks of energy and can usually find a way for you to figure out the solution for yourself.

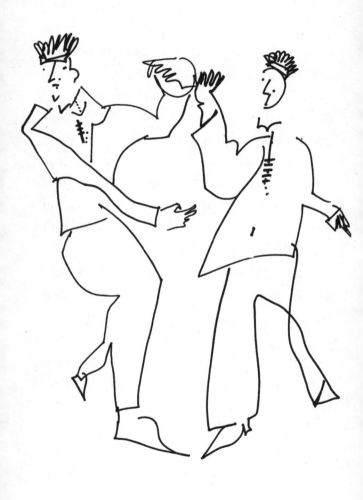

86 There is no good or bad Chi, just Chi. It is always subjective to where you are, at the moment. Beneficial or detrimental would be a better way to think about it. A drop of water in an empty glass would start to fill it (beneficial). A drop of water in a full glass would overflow it (detrimental). That idea gives us more personal responsibility for our lives and actions.

87 The eight cranial bones of the skull are capable of minute movements. This movement is important to pump the cerebrospinal fluid which surrounds and nourishes the brain and the spinal cord. We can increase the movements of the joints of the cranium and increase the function of the pumping action of the cranial pump. Use your mind to do this. When inhaling, imagine the skull expanding, and when exhaling, allow the skull to relax. After practicing this for a while, make sure to ground the energy in order to balance it and keep you from getting top heavy. To ground

81

the energy, imagine the energy coming in through the Bai Hui point on the top of the head, and moving down through the body and out through the bottoms of the feet.

88 When one part of the body moves, every part moves. Push a ball anywhere and see what happens. Visualize your body as a ball with your Dan Tien at the center of the ball. Keep your attention in your Dan Tien as you move and your movements will take on a real sense of beauty brought about by the unification of a structure in motion.

89 Tai Chi weapons practice isn't about learning how to cut someone up with a sword or saber. The most important lessons have to do with learning the ability to lead Chi or energy into an object. We need this skill in order to hit a baseball or golf ball or tennis ball. We need this skill in order to use a pen or pencil or paint brush. Think about a toothbrush, a knife, a screwdriver, a steering wheel, or bicycle. Every object that we use requires an interaction between us and it, and how we do this will determine much about our health and happiness. We need to learn how to do the most with the least expenditure of energy, and in the case of most sports, how to transfer the greatest amount of energy into the object we are working with. So look for the opportunity to study Tai Chi weapons and you'll certainly improve the quality of your life.

90 That which is strong will always end up losing to the weak, the high gives to the low, the full to the empty. That is the way of the Tao. Water will always seek the lowest level. Hot and cold air will seek a common temperature. If you want to be filled, first you must empty. If you want to receive, giving will make it possible. If you want to be loved, make sure you can give your love. The universe is very clear on these principles.

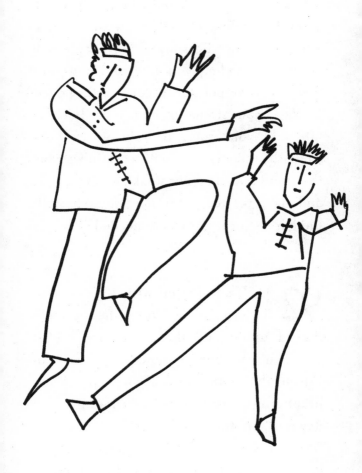

91 It is always a good idea to conceal your power. Don't show that which you value and people will not want to take it away from you. Be simple and people will always want to help you. In Push Hands, this idea is very important. If your partner doesn't know your strengths, he is more likely to fall into your trap. If he can see your strengths clearly, he will certainly avoid them and seek out your weakness. Be simple and open, yet keep your most valuable skills hidden until they are truly needed.

92 Drill an oil well with your coccyx. This means to keep the buttocks tucked under and the spine erect. That way you can bob up and down without interfering with your alignment. When practicing your forms, bounce up and down when the weight is on the rear or front foot or between to test yourself. If you can bounce, it means that the energy is moving to the floor and back up and not getting stuck in the joints. Try locking your knee joint and then try bouncing and you'll see what I mean.

93 Tai Chi stepping is like walking on a newly frozen lake. Test the ground when you place the stepping foot before committing all your weight. You want to be able to withdraw at anytime without jerking your body back. It is the same with stepping backwards. And keep in mind that most of the time you are stepping to the side and to the rear of your opponent, so place your foot accordingly. Never lose control of the weight of the body when stepping. Watch most people walk and you will notice that they are constantly falling forward and their feet keep moving to keep them from falling on their face. Set your foot first, then move onto it.

94 There is a magic place in New Zealand called Pou-Pou Springs. Out of a hole in the ground, about 30 feet in diameter, gushes crystal clear water that is the start of a fairly large river. It is amazing to see that much water come out of a hole in the ground. Keeping the Spring in my mind has helped my Tai Chi practice many times. I imagine that Pou-Pou Springs is located in my belly, and water (energy) rushes out into places my mind directs in a powerful, never ending stream. It works for me, so it might work for you if you try it yourself.

95 Open, loosen, and relax are three words that are very important to keep our joints and body healthy. Always keep the idea of these when doing any movement. For instance, many people are told not to do neck rolls, as it is commonly believed that this movement can injure the neck. First off, I believe that if the body can do a movement, like roll the neck, we should continue to do the movement very gently, but also to its maximum. If we don't, stiffness might set in and we won't be able to do as full a movement. It is like a hinge.

If it is not used, it gets rusty and then can't work. So if you keep the idea of open, loosen and relax in mind when gently rolling the neck, you'll get nothing but benefit. Also, do these in order, first open, then loosen, and finally relax.

96 Buckminister Fuller, one of the true geniuses of our time, once said that, in proportion, we have more space between each cell of our body than there is between each star in the galaxy. When we look at our body, we see solid mass, and when we look toward the sky, we see mostly space. Assuming Buckminister was correct, this knowledge can help us a great deal in our Tai Chi practice. Allow the spaces to enlarge in order to gain a feeling of being light and agile. Flexibility will be enhanced, as will the skill of joining with someone. It is easy to allow energy in and out when there is a feeling of space. Let your breath open your spaces. Relax and let the universe move through you.

97 It has been said that play is where cognition and culture meet. Play might be our most important thinking tool, particularly when we are learning to think in new ways. Push Hands is play on so many levels, and we can learn the basic and classic teachings about Tai Chi Chuan, especially if we don't approach Push Hands with the need to always win. Watching young animals play is a good lesson on learning serious survival skills through a more light hearted approach. So, play Tai Chi and you'll reap the benefits with a smile on your face.

98 You can only push something. This means you must be able to recognize substantial and insubstantial. Do not try and push if you do not feel tension in your opponent. Set it up first if you must by faking. Make him start to move. You want him to be over extended and to move into your strong centered place. Be like a spider and wait for him to enter your web.

99 The study of Tai Chi Chuan is the study of our essential nature. This Real You is at the center of your being, alive yet covered by layers of illusion that shield Reality from view. The fabric of illusion is made of expectations from our parents and society, self delusion, fear, and poor habits. Tai Chi helps to shed the layers, starting from the outside, or physical, and moving inward toward the energetic and spiritual. First the physical is examined for any non essential elements, mostly tension, which are then eliminated. The body is strengthened and relaxed. The second layer is the energetic body which is examined by the study and practice of Chi Kung, using breath and visualization to open to and gain control of Chi or energy. The energy is then refined and focused. The deepest layer or that of our true or spiritual nature is experienced by meditation. The physical body and energetic body have been opened, strengthened, and now the final barrier to self knowledge will fall through the practice of mindfulness training or meditation. All spiritual traditions, including Tai Chi and Taoism, use this sequence to gain awareness of the True Self. Look to those that have gone before and listen to their advice. Then eliminate that which doesn't work, or what your intuition tells you isn't right for you. There are no short cuts, so use your time wisely and stay on the path. Keep a smile on your face and be thankful you have the opportunity to discover your True Self and how it relates to the Universe.

100

The ideal time for your Tai Chi practice is in the early morning as the sun is rising. The energy is quite pure, the Yang Chi is growing, yet it is still cool and quiet. Tai Chi as a healthy exercise needs to be practiced on a daily basis, and it is easier to make time before you get your busy day started then sometime in the midst of it. Your day will always go more smoothly when you are relaxed, energized, and centered. So, get up a few minutes earlier each day, do your Tai Chi, and you'll notice after a short while how much better you are feeling.

101 Stop, Look, and Listen. Stop means to still the mind. Look means to observe the opponent without prejudice or fear. Listen means to incorporate all your senses, especially your touch, into understanding the energy of your opponent.

102 Energy moves only because there are differences between one point and another. We must embrace difference because difference gives movement and movement gives life.

103 As you progress in your studies of Tai Chi, you will start to feel various sensations as the energy starts to move into and through the body. It is important to view these as sensations, not pleasure or pain. If we think pleasure and pain, we will seek one and reject the other, and that will most assuredly cause us to miss the reality of the moment. Examine very closely each body sensation in order to gain an understanding of how the body works and how it is put together. Energy is energy, and as it moves through the body it will interact with your structure in such a way as to cause a sensation. As you get more sensitive, you will be able to detect more subtle forms of energy. The whole idea of Tai Chi as a healing art and martial art is to get so sensitive to the movement of Chi that we can tell if it starts to get too Yin or too Yang, and be able to deal with it before it gets too far out of balance. Every big problem started out small, so examine yourself closely on a daily basis through the practice of Tai Chi and you will keep yourself healthy.

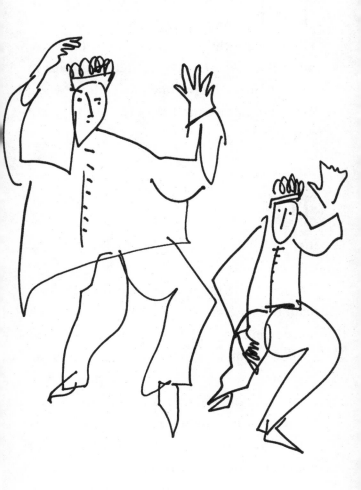

104 The body of the Tai Chi practitioner is like a horse and rider. The legs are the horse, the upper body the rider. It is important to separate the rider so he can turn around and do actions while the horse does something else, yet they are one unit.

105 Energy follows the mind, so make sure to have the eyes involved in every movement of Tai Chi. The eyes generally slightly lead the movement of the body, in order to assess the situation and lead the energy. Fast movement is much more accurately picked up with peripheral vision, so don't try and focus directly on the incoming energy, but glance slightly to the side. When following your own hand movements, glance about a foot beyond your active hand because that is where your opponent would be. Also when working with a partner or doing your solo form, perform as if there were someone there and keep your eyes mostly on the other person's center. All effective movement comes from the center, so you'll be able to pick up movement before it has a chance to move to the arms and hands and build up power. The eyes express the spirit, so if you want to relax, let the eyes relax and glance in front of the body at a 45 degree angle downward. If you want to be like a tiger, open the eyes wider and let that tiger energy be alive in your eyes.

106 There is no such thing as retreat (in the usual sense people tend to think about it) in Tai Chi. When faced with a powerful force, we sometimes withdraw into a new position with the idea of leading our opponent into a trap. Once the opponent starts to follow me, he is more exposed to counter attack, especially on his flanks or sides. The Tai Chi movement "Step Back and Repulse Monkey" is a clear illustration of this principle. The opponent makes a strong attack toward my center with his right fist. I step back with my right foot, join his incoming energy with my right hand, and lead it to my right side into nothingness. My opponent is now in big trouble. Not only is he quite exposed and most probably out of his center as a result of my leading his forward momentum further then he wanted to go, but also I have successfully closed up his ability to attack further by drawing his forward arm (his right) across his body. I can now use my left hand to attack his right side, which lies exposed.

107 The earliest movements upon which Tai Chi was based were the Five Animal Frolics. The animals are the tiger, bear, stork, deer, and monkey. Each of these animals has its own unique energy, and these various energies can make your Tai Chi practice interesting and fun if you explore them. Think about one of these animals and how it moves and acts. Then do a form and see if you can express this particular energy throughout. After you have played with the original Five Animals, experiment with other animals like the snake, reptile, fish, etc. Then try a tree, a rock, water, air, or anything you can imagine. Your form will grow, expand, enliven, and bring you much joy, pleasure, and spiritual wonder.

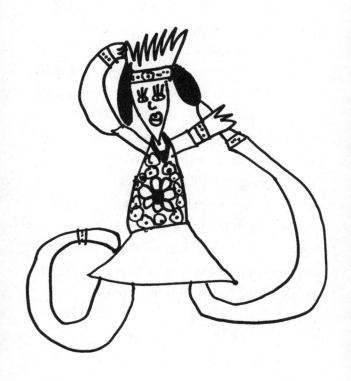

Drawing by Azzura Lockwood, age 5.

108 The most powerful martial art is meditation. If we have a calm, relaxed mind, we will be able to see clearly and be able to deal with situations before they build up to a point of no return. Only when you stake out a position and decide to stay there are you vulnerable to being pushed over. Water will move out of the way, yet doesn't lose its essential nature. If you freeze or heat water, it will adapt to the new situation and then return to normal when the pressure is off. If we let go of our ego and let go of thinking about ourselves as we used to be, we will be able to be reborn each moment into a new person, comprised of our essential nature.

Glossary of Terms

These are some of the terms I used in this book that might not be familiar to everybody. I am assuming that anybody reading this book has at least some knowledge of Tai Chi Chuan and the terms associated with its study, yet with the many different spellings and translations of Chinese terms, I want you to be clear about what I mean.

Bai Hui

The opening at the top of the head where Yang Chi or cosmic Chi enters and leaves the body. Sometimes referred to as the Crown Chakra.

Chi Energy

Generally refers to the energy that moves through the universe and also through man. Chi is the battery that drives all life. Shen is the most refined Chi and Jieng is the grossest.

Chi Kung

Energy exercises or breathing exercises. There are thousands of general and specific exercises to build energy or Chi. Tai Chi Chuan could be considered an elaborate Chi Kung exercise.

Dan Tien

Storage vessel for acquired energy, usually referring to the lower Dan Tien located slightly below the navel. In Tai Chi and many forms of Chi Kung, the mind is centered on the Dan Tien, thereby moving energy that is acquired into that storage site to be used or refined.

Hsin

Heart mind. The emotional and feeling part of our mind, usually thought to reside in the heart.

Hui Yin

Gate of life and death. The perineum or floor of the pelvis. The meeting place for the Yin energy as it rises up the two legs.

Jieng

Essential Chi. This is the Chi or energy that is given to us at birth. It is genetic, potential energy and is limited in quantity for most people. The Taoists have practices for turning Chi and Jieng into Shen.

Jing

The expression of energy. Usually refers to how energy is expressed. There are hundreds of different Jings, including Fa Jing which is an explosive burst of energy used in Push Hands and fighting.

Kua

The inguinal fold or front of the groin. It is important to have flexibility in this area in order to gather energy there for later release. It is the area used to crouch.

Lao Kung

An opening in the center of each palm for energy to enter and leave the body.

Macrocosmic Orbit:

Important for Tai Chi players in that the energy orbit not only goes up the back and down the front, but also moves into the arms.

Microcosmic Orbit

The circular pathway for the movement of energy in the body. Basically, up the back, over the head, and down the front. There are many blocks or gates along the path that have to opened so the energy can pass through. Tai Chi, Chi Kung and many other forms of meditative energy work utilize the idea of moving energy around this orbit.

Ming Men

Door of Life. The storage place for prenatal Chi or the energy given to us at birth. Located between the kidneys.

Push Hands

An important training device used in Tai Chi Chuan. It involves two people, usually in fixed position, giving and receiving energy, using Tai Chi movements and principles, with the intention of developing an awareness of the highest levels of Tai Chi. There are competitions in Push Hands where each person tries to uproot and make the other person lose balance.

Shen

The highest and most refined form of energy with which man interacts. When the Shen is cultivated and focused, the blocks to man's realization of the Tao can be dissolved. Tai Chi Chuan uses Shen to reach the highest skill levels.

Tao and Taoism

Tao is all-inclusive everythingness. It is beyond understanding, yet can be experienced. Taoism is the study of Tao and how man can let go of his separate ego and reunite with this universal energy.

Tai Chi

Used as a shortened version of Tai Chi Chuan, or can mean the state of balance between Yin and Yang before they seperate.

Tai Chi Chuan

The name of an internal martial art developed in China. It means the form or

Wu Chi

The state of perfect balance where there is no movement. The state before the forming of the universe, before the appearance of Yin and Yang.

Yi

The conscious mind. The thinking and reasoning part of our brain.

Yin and Yang

The complimentary opposites. These are the expressions of how energy is manifesting at the moment to a specific observer. Yin and Yang are each given various qualities that signify opposition or balance. There has to be Yin to have Yang, night to have day, soft to have hard, in to have out, down to have up, cool to have hot, female to have male, etc. We have to be clear that all of these are only relative terms. There is not absolute hot, or up, or in. A tree may be harder than water, yet softer than a rock.

Yung Chuan

The opening at the bottom of the foot for the Yin Chi or earth energy to enter and leave the body. This is an accupoint, K-1, the start of the kidney meridian.

About the Author

Michael Gilman, a long time teacher in the human potential movement, was born in San Francisco in 1943. After graduating from the University of Arizona with a degree in Theatre Arts, he worked as a television director, actor, and dancer.

Gilman began his studies of Tai Chi Chuan in 1968 with Master Choy Kam-Man in San Francisco. Master Choy's father, Choy Hok Peng, a long time student of Yang Chen Fu, is credited with introducing Tai Chi to America in the 1940's. Master Choy taught the full traditional Yang Style Tai Chi curriculum, and that is the system that Michael still practices and teaches.

Michael was authorized to teach by Master Choy in 1973 and moved to Tucson, Arizona to begin teaching. Over most of the next eight years, Michael worked with over a thousand people, including such diverse groups as the Tucson Ballet Co., Tucson Opera, Tucson Museum of Art, University of Arizona, Tucson Public Schools, YMCA, as well as running a successful Tai Chi Studio. During this period he also taught in Florida, Oregon, California and New Zealand.

In 1981, Michael moved to Port Townsend, Washington, and opened his Studio where he currently teaches. He also teaches many workshops. Besides his long term association with Master Choy, Michael has studied Tai Chi with Jou Tsung Hwa, Dr. Yang, Jwing-Ming, T.Y. Pang, T.T. Liang, George Xu, William Chen, Liang, Shou-Yu, Tao Ping-Siang, Fu Shen Yuan, Gao Fu, Ken Cohen, and Sam Masich.

In 1994, Michael won the title of Grand Champion at the prestigious "A Taste of China" All Tai Chi Tournament in Virginia. In 1995, he was honored by being chosen as an advanced form judge of Internal Arts at the International Kung Fu Championships in Seattle.

In addition to *A String of Pearls*, Michael has been published in Tai Chi Magazine, written *The Tai Chi Manual*, and has produced various video tapes. He has been much honored for his work with teenagers.

Michael's eclectic interests, study and teaching include Advita Yoga with Master Subramuniya (Michael was Master Subramuniya's personal chef), Hatha Yoga with Swami Vishnudevananda (Michael taught Yoga at Vishnudevananda ashram), Zen Buddhism, Arica (Michael taught in Tucson), Trager Psychophysical Integration (taught for the Trager Institute) and Dependable Strengths (Michael teaches for the Dependable Strengths Institute).

Michael has also spent much of the past few years developing a new exercise system to complement Tai Chi, and is currently working on a book and video teaching the system.

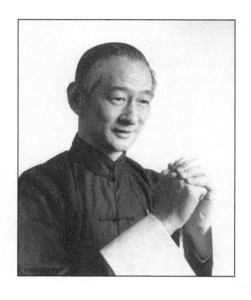

To the memory of Master Choy Kam Man
(1924-1994)

His father, Choy Hok Peng (1885-1958) is
considered to be the father of Tai Chi in America